Diabetes Management: The Role of Physical Activity and Medicinal Plants

Dr. Alireza Barari,

Mahboubeh Khak Rand

Dr. Asieh Abbassi Daloii

Diabetes Management: The Role of Physical Activity and Medicinal Plants

ISBN: 978-1-962443-12-8

THE CONCEPTS THAT USED IN THIS BOOK ARE A SELECTION OF THE BASIC CONCEPTS OF DIABETES AND PHYSICAL ACTIVITY THAT CAN BE USEFUL FOR ALL PEOPLE AND PEOPLES THAT INTERESTED IN SPORTS. WE DEDICATE THIS CONTENT TO FMILIES.

CONTENTS

CHAPTER 1: Diabetes

Diabetes is a metabolic disorder characterized by elevated blood glucose levels. It results from a defect in insulin secretion, reduced sensitivity of glucose receptors in cells, or a combination of both.

Types of Diabetes

Diabetes is classified into several types, the most common being:

1. **Type 1 Diabetes**
2. **Type 2 Diabetes**
3. **Gestational Diabetes**

Type 1 Diabetes

Type 1 diabetes, also known as insulin-dependent diabetes mellitus (IDDM), is caused by insufficient insulin production. It typically manifests before the age of 40 and is therefore referred to as juvenile diabetes. Individuals with type 1 diabetes are usually not obese, but they are more prone to conditions like ketosis and acidosis.

A key characteristic of type 1 diabetes is the presence of anti-B-cell antibodies in the blood plasma, though it is now understood that the disease is primarily mediated by T-type lymphocytes. Genetic predisposition plays a significant role, with the major genetic defect linked to the major histocompatibility complex (MHC) on chromosome 6.

Type 2 Diabetes

Type 2 diabetes is a prevalent metabolic disease affecting an estimated 5-8% of adults globally. In 2010, 285 million people were diagnosed with type 2 diabetes, and this number is projected to reach 438 million by 2030. Individuals with type 2 diabetes are at twice the risk of premature death, cardiovascular disease, kidney disease, neurological disorders, and blindness compared to non-diabetics.

Blood Glucose Levels

- Normal fasting blood glucose: 70–99 mg/dL
- Prediabetes: 100–125 mg/dL
- Diabetes: >126 mg/dL

Prediabetes, a precursor to type 2 diabetes, occurs when blood glucose levels are slightly elevated but not yet high enough to be classified as diabetes. Without intervention, prediabetes often progresses to type 2 diabetes.

Causes and Mechanisms

Type 2 diabetes, also known as non-insulin-dependent diabetes mellitus (NIDDM), is primarily caused by reduced sensitivity of target tissues to insulin—a condition known as insulin resistance. Obesity is the most significant risk factor, with increased prevalence in both adults and children due to lifestyle changes.

Key features of type 2 diabetes include:

- Gradual onset, often after age 30, though increasing rates in children are linked to obesity.
- Hyperinsulinemia (elevated insulin levels) as a compensatory response to insulin resistance.
- Rare association with ketosis.
- Genetic factors, including over 60 identified gene mutations, such as defects in glucokinase, insulin receptors, and GLUT4.

Impact on Metabolism

Both type 1 and type 2 diabetes disrupt the metabolism of carbohydrates, fats, and proteins. Insufficient insulin or insulin resistance impairs glucose uptake by most cells (except brain cells), leading to hyperglycemia. In response, the body increases fat and protein utilization as alternative energy sources.

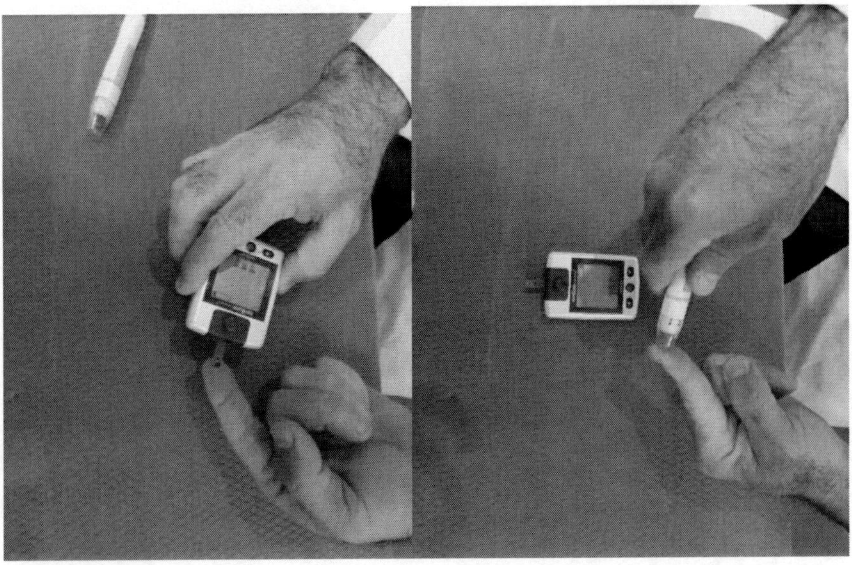

Figure 1: Blood Glucose Measurement by Glucometer

Diabetes Mellitus

Diabetes mellitus is a syndrome characterized by disturbances in the metabolism of carbohydrates, fats, and proteins. These disruptions result from either insufficient insulin secretion or decreased tissue sensitivity to insulin.

While the majority of diabetes cases fall under the categories of type 1, type 2, or gestational diabetes, some types stem from other underlying conditions. These are often referred to as **secondary diabetes** and account for about 5% of all diabetes cases. Causes of secondary diabetes include:

- Chronic pancreatitis
- Surgical removal of the pancreas

- Cushing's syndrome
- Acromegaly

Gestational Diabetes (Pregnancy)

Gestational diabetes occurs during pregnancy and usually resolves after the baby is born. During pregnancy, the placenta produces hormones essential for the growth and development of the fetus. However, these hormones can interfere with the mother's insulin action, leading to increased insulin requirements—up to two or three times higher than normal.

When the mother's body cannot produce sufficient insulin to meet this increased demand, gestational diabetes develops. Testing for gestational diabetes is typically conducted between the **24th and 28th weeks of pregnancy**.

Gestational diabetes may recur in subsequent pregnancies, and if blood sugar levels remain elevated, it can lead to complications such as:

- **Macrosomia**: Excessive growth of the baby, which can make delivery more difficult.
- Increased risk of the baby developing diabetes later in life.

CHAPTER 2: Complications of Diabetes

Diabetes has minimal immediate effects in its early stages, but as the disease progresses, it can severely impact vital organs, including the heart, blood vessels, nerves, kidneys, and eyes. Proper blood sugar control is crucial to preventing these complications.

Common Complications of Diabetes

1. **Cardiovascular Disease (CVD)**
   Diabetes significantly increases the risk of cardiovascular diseases, including:
   - Coronary artery disease (CAD) with symptoms such as chest pain (angina)
   - Heart attack
   - Stroke
   - Atherosclerosis
   - High blood pressure
2. **Nerve Damage (Neuropathy)**
   Elevated blood sugar levels can damage the blood vessels supplying the nerves, particularly in the legs and feet. This can result in:
   - Numbness
   - Burning sensations
   - Pain in fingers and toes

3. **Kidney Damage (Nephropathy)**
   Diabetes can damage the delicate blood vessels within the kidneys, impairing their function. Left untreated, this may lead to kidney failure or the need for dialysis.

4. **Eye Damage (Retinopathy)**
   High blood sugar can harm the blood vessels in the retina, potentially leading to:
   - Diabetic retinopathy, which may result in blindness
   - Cataracts
   - Glaucoma

5. **Foot Complications**
   Nerve damage and reduced blood flow to the feet can lead to severe foot infections or ulcers. In extreme cases, this may result in toe or limb amputation.

6. **Skin and Oral Issues**
   Diabetes increases the risk of skin infections, fungal infections, and oral conditions such as gum disease and pus formation in the throat.

7. **Alzheimer's Disease**
   Type 2 diabetes has been linked to a higher risk of Alzheimer's disease, possibly due to the effects of insulin resistance on the brain.

8. **Diabetic Coma**
   Severe dehydration or prolonged high blood sugar levels can

lead to diabetic coma, a life-threatening condition.

9. **Other Complications**
    - **Hearing Problems**: Diabetes can damage the auditory nerves, leading to hearing loss.
    - **Osteoporosis**: Long-term diabetes may reduce bone density, increasing fracture risks.

Cardiovascular Disease (CVD)

CVD is an umbrella term for diseases involving the heart and blood vessels. This includes:

- **Coronary Heart Disease (CHD)**: Narrowing or blockage of coronary arteries due to plaque buildup.
- **Coronary Artery Disease (CAD)**: Characterized by atherosclerosis in coronary arteries, which can lead to reduced blood flow.
- **Acute Coronary Syndrome (ACS)**: Usually symptomatic and associated with unstable angina or myocardial infarction (heart attack).

Risk Factors for CVD

CVD is largely preventable, but its prevalence is increasing due to:

- Physical inactivity

- Smoking
- Poor dietary habits

Atherosclerosis and Coronary Heart Disease

Atherosclerosis refers to the formation of plaques composed of cholesterol, fat, calcium, and other substances within the walls of arteries. It reduces blood flow and can lead to:

- **Cardiovascular Disease (CVD)**: Affects the heart and peripheral blood vessels.
- **Cerebrovascular Disease**: Can cause ischemic strokes in the brain.

Coronary Artery Disease (CAD) occurs when these plaques block blood flow in the coronary arteries, reducing oxygen supply to the heart muscle. This can result in:

- **Angina** (chest pain) caused by restricted blood flow
- Heart attack if oxygen supply is severely reduced

Lifestyle and CVD Prevention

Studies show that high consumption of saturated fats and physical inactivity significantly increase the risk of cardiovascular diseases. Inactivity leads to weight gain, high blood pressure, and increased cholesterol levels, all of which contribute to atherosclerosis.

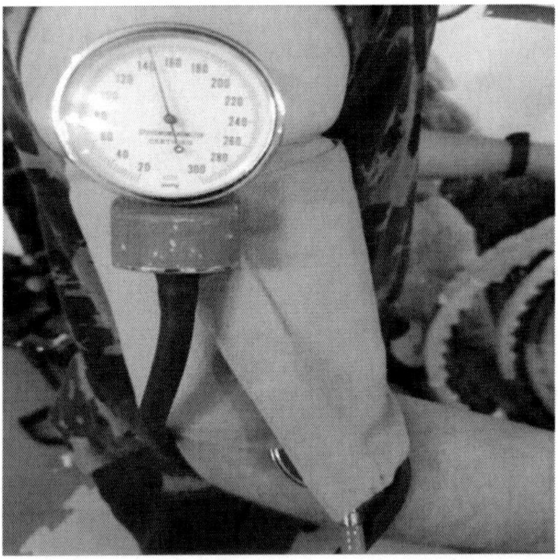

Figure 2: Blood Pressure Measurement Using a Sphygmomanometer.

Recent studies have observed that physical activity can improve cardiorespiratory function and that physical inactivity is a modifiable risk factor for the development of atherosclerosis.

Diabetes, if not well-managed, can cause severe complications over time. These complications often affect vital organs and bodily systems, such as the cardiovascular system, kidneys, and eyes. Early detection and management are essential to reduce risks. Below are detailed discussions of major diabetes-related complications.

Common Tests to Diagnose Heart Failure

Myocardial infarction (MI), or heart attack, is the ischemic necrosis of heart muscle tissue caused by a blood supply obstruction. This often occurs due to the formation of atherosclerotic plaques, which result from the gradual accumulation of cholesterol and fats under the arterial walls. Over time, these deposits harden into calcified plaques, which can partially or fully block coronary arteries, restricting blood flow to the heart.

Causes of Acute Coronary Occlusion

1. **Plaque Rupture**: Leads to the aggregation of platelets, red blood cells, and fibrin, forming a thrombus that obstructs blood flow.
2. **Coronary Artery Spasm**: Caused by:
   - Stimulation of the coronary artery wall.
   - Local nerve reflexes causing vasoconstriction and thrombosis.

When coronary arteries are blocked, heart muscle cells die due to oxygen deprivation, leading to myocardial infarction. This process causes cell swelling, leakage of cellular contents, and eventual tissue edema.

Clinical Symptoms of Myocardial Infarction

1. Chest pain, increased breathing rate, and shortened breathing duration.
2. Reduced cardiac output, which can lead to cardiogenic shock.
3. Accumulation of blood in pulmonary veins, resulting in pulmonary edema.
4. Ventricular fibrillation and severe heart damage.

Laboratory Diagnostic Tests for Myocardial Infarction

Laboratory tests play a crucial role in diagnosing heart attacks. Commonly evaluated biomarkers include:

1. **Creatine Kinase (CK or CPK)**
   - **CK-MB**: A specific isozyme for heart tissue.
     - Increases within 3-6 hours post-MI.
     - Peaks at 12-24 hours and normalizes in 12-48 hours.

- Useful for diagnosing myocardial infarction, but it lacks sensitivity due to overlap with skeletal muscle injury.

2. **Myoglobin**
   - An oxygen-binding protein useful for early MI detection.
   - Increases about 3 hours after cardiac muscle damage.
   - Highly sensitive but not specific, as it also rises with skeletal muscle injuries.
3. **Troponin (cTnI and cTnT)**
   - Highly specific markers for cardiac muscle injury.
   - Levels rise 2-3 hours after injury and remain elevated for 7-14 days.
   - More sensitive and specific than CK-MB.
4. **Lactate Dehydrogenase (LDH)**
   - Increases 24-48 hours after MI, peaks at 2-3 days, and normalizes within 5-10 days.
   - Useful for late-stage MI diagnosis, but less specific compared to troponin tests.

Diabetes and Kidney Disease

Diabetic nephropathy, or diabetic kidney disease (DKD), is a common long-term complication of diabetes. High blood sugar levels can damage the glomeruli in the kidneys, impairing their filtration function.

Key Features

- Leakage of proteins, especially albumin, into the urine (proteinuria).

- Increased risk of kidney failure, where waste products like urea and creatinine accumulate in the blood.

Symptoms of Kidney Failure

- Swelling in the ankles, face, or abdomen.
- Fatigue, weakness, and confusion.
- Loss of appetite, vomiting, and headaches.

Contributing Factors

- Persistent hyperglycemia.
- High blood pressure.
- Genetic predisposition.

Diabetes and Eye Diseases

Chronic high blood sugar can damage various parts of the eye, leading to vision impairment or loss.

Diabetic Retinopathy

Occurs when high blood sugar damages retinal blood vessels, leading to:

- Swelling and leakage of retinal blood vessels.
- Blocked blood flow to the retina.
- Formation of fragile new blood vessels, which may bleed into the vitreous humor, causing vision problems or blindness.

Diabetes and Cataracts

Cataracts result from the destruction of lens proteins, making the lens opaque.

- **Symptoms**:
    - Blurred vision.
    - Double vision (diplopia).
    - Increased sensitivity to light.
    - Difficulty seeing in low light.

Diabetes and Glaucoma

Glaucoma is characterized by increased intraocular pressure, damaging the optic nerve. Diabetes doubles the risk of developing glaucoma due to impaired drainage of intraocular fluid. If untreated, this condition can cause irreversible vision loss.

CHAPTER 3: Diabetes and Metabolic Indices

Diabetes, Inflammatory Indicators, and Exercise

Diabetes is a chronic metabolic disorder characterized by a relative deficiency or absence of insulin in the bloodstream. This leads to persistently high blood glucose levels and an accumulation of glycosylated substances, increasing the risk of cardiovascular disease. One of the hallmark features of diabetes is **systemic mild chronic inflammation**.

Inflammatory Mediators in Diabetes

Patients with diabetes often exhibit elevated levels of inflammatory mediators, such as cytokines and C-reactive protein (CRP). These markers play a significant role in the development and progression of cardiovascular complications associated with diabetes. Key inflammatory cytokines include:

1. **Interleukin-1 (IL-1)**
2. **Tumor Necrosis Factor-Alpha (TNF-α)**
3. **Interleukin-6 (IL-6)**

These cytokines trigger a cascade of inflammatory reactions, leading to the secretion of additional mediators like:

- **C-Reactive Protein (CRP)**
- **Interleukin-8 (IL-8)**
- **Intercellular Adhesion Molecule-1 (ICAM-1)**

This inflammatory process disrupts insulin signaling pathways, reducing insulin sensitivity and exacerbating hyperglycemia.

The Role of Physical Activity

Physical activity has been shown to exert both preventive and therapeutic effects against diabetes and its associated complications. One of its primary benefits is the reduction of systemic inflammation, which is achieved through various mechanisms:

1. **Reduction in Body Fat**:
    - Physical activity increases lipolysis (fat breakdown), reducing adipose tissue—a significant source of inflammatory mediators.
2. **Improved Insulin Sensitivity**:
    - Regular exercise enhances insulin signaling and glucose uptake, mitigating inflammation-related insulin resistance.
3. **Enhanced Physical Fitness**:
    - Higher levels of physical fitness are consistently associated with lower levels of inflammatory markers such as CRP and IL-6.

Evidence from Research

Studies consistently demonstrate that physical activity reduces systemic inflammation, regardless of diabetes status. Endurance and resistance training, in particular, are effective in promoting anti-inflammatory responses and improving metabolic health.

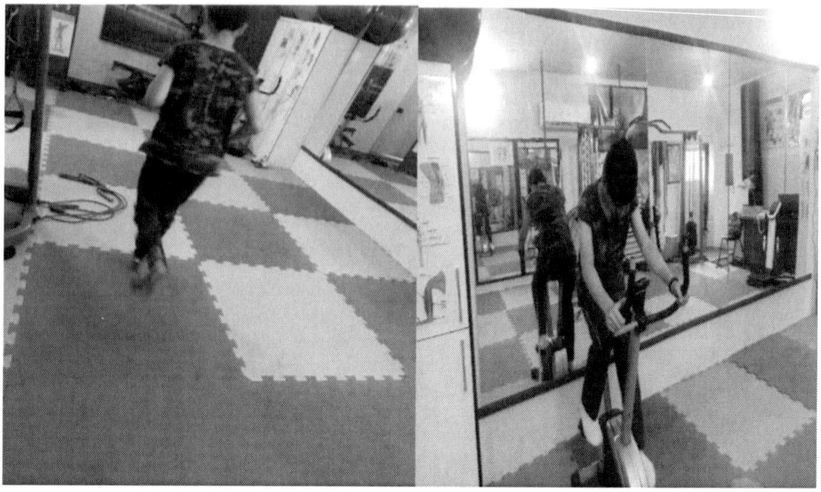

Figure 3: Body’s Physiological Responses to Endurance Training

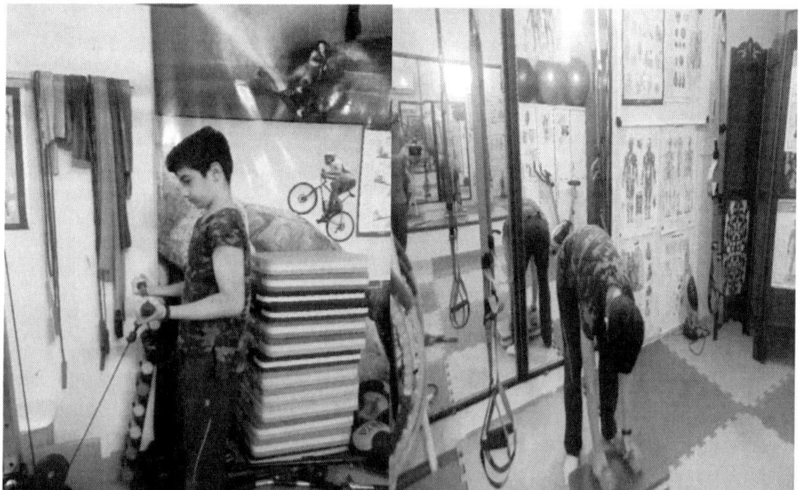

Figure4. body's Physiological Adaptations by resistance training

Type 2 Diabetes and Decreased Metabolic Effects of Insulin

Role of Insulin in Glucose Metabolism

In mammals, insulin is the primary hormone responsible for regulating blood glucose levels. It facilitates glucose uptake into cells, boosts metabolism in muscle and fat tissues, and inhibits gluconeogenesis (the production of glucose) in the liver.

Discovery of Insulin

The discovery and synthesis of insulin in 1921 by Sir Frederick Grant Banting and Charles Herbert Best revolutionized diabetes treatment, allowing individuals with type 1 diabetes to live relatively normal lives.

Structure and Function

- **Insulin** is a polypeptide hormone secreted by the beta cells in the islets of Langerhans in the pancreas.
- It comprises 51 amino acids with a molecular weight of 5,808 daltons.
- Insulin biosynthesis involves the production of **preinsulin**, which is rapidly converted into insulin and **C-peptide**.

Insulin Secretion

Pancreatic beta cells have a high capacity to store insulin, which can constitute up to 10% of their protein volume. Insulin secretion occurs in two phases:

1. **First Phase**: A rapid release of stored insulin occurs in response to elevated glucose levels shortly after a meal, lasting about 6 minutes.
2. **Second Phase**: Sustained secretion of insulin over 10-13 minutes to maintain low blood glucose levels.

When insulin is absent or ineffective, glucose is not absorbed by cells, forcing the body to rely on fat as an energy source.

Insulin Resistance

Definition and Mechanism

Insulin resistance is a condition in which cells fail to respond adequately to insulin, impairing glucose absorption and leading to elevated blood sugar levels. Although the pancreas produces sufficient or even excessive amounts of insulin, the cells' response to it is diminished.

Key Features

1. **Obesity as a Trigger**:
    - Obesity, particularly excess fat accumulation in tissues such as skeletal muscle and liver, is a major contributor to insulin resistance.
    - Studies suggest that obese individuals have fewer insulin receptors in their skeletal muscle, liver, and fat tissues compared to those with normal weight.
2. **Impact on Glucose Regulation**:
    - Normally, insulin suppresses glucose release from liver cells. In insulin resistance, this suppression fails, leading to elevated blood glucose levels.
    - Fat and muscle cells also exhibit impaired glucose uptake.
3. **Connection to Obesity**:
    - Obesity exacerbates insulin resistance, making it a key risk factor for type 2 diabetes.
    - It leads to hyperinsulinemia (elevated insulin levels), dyslipidemia (abnormal lipid levels), and impaired glucose tolerance.

Pathophysiological Effects

Insulin resistance contributes to a range of metabolic disorders, including:

- Hypertension
- Dyslipidemia
- Cardiovascular disease
- Type 2 diabetes

Role of Adipose Tissue

Adipose tissue plays a significant role in insulin resistance through the irregular production of various proteins, including:

- Tumor Necrosis Factor-Alpha (TNF-α)
- Leptin
- Adiponectin
- Angiotensin
- Resistin

Measurement of Insulin Resistance

The **HOMA-IR (Homeostatic Model Assessment of Insulin Resistance)** index is a common tool for evaluating insulin resistance. It provides insights into the balance between insulin secretion and insulin sensitivity.

CHAPTER 4: Diabetes Diagnosis

The accurate diagnosis of diabetes relies heavily on laboratory criteria. According to the American Diabetes Association (ADA), a definitive diagnosis of diabetes can only be established through clinical laboratory tests. Among these, the **Hemoglobin A1c (HbA1c)** test has emerged as one of the most important diagnostic tools.

Diagnostic Criteria for Type 2 Diabetes

The ADA recognizes the following four diagnostic methods for diabetes:

1. **Hemoglobin A1c (HbA1c) Test**
    - Measures the amount of glucose attached to hemoglobin in red blood cells.
    - A result of HbA1c ≥ 6.5% indicates diabetes.
2. **Fasting Plasma Glucose (FPG)**
    - Measures blood sugar after fasting for at least 8 hours.
    - A fasting blood glucose level of **≥126 mg/dL** confirms diabetes.
3. **Oral Glucose Tolerance Test (OGTT)**
    - Measures blood sugar in two states: fasting and 2 hours after consuming 75 grams of glucose.
        - A result of **140–199 mg/dL** at 2 hours indicates **pre-diabetes**.
        - A result of **≥200 mg/dL** at 2 hours confirms diabetes.
4. **Random Plasma Glucose Test**
    - Measures blood glucose levels at any time, regardless of

meal timing.

- A glucose level of **≥200 mg/dL** in the presence of hyperglycemic symptoms (e.g., polyuria, polydipsia, weight loss) confirms diabetes.

Important Considerations

1. **Fasting Period**:
   - While the recommended fasting period is at least 8 hours, some guidelines suggest a range of 8–14 hours. However, fasting beyond 14 hours may not be practical or necessary.
2. **Repeat Testing**:
   - In the absence of hyperglycemic symptoms, a second test on a different day is required to confirm the diagnosis.
3. **Standard Conditions for Glucose Tolerance Test**:
   - Conducted after at least 3 days of an unrestricted diet (≥150 grams of carbohydrates daily) and normal physical activity.

Glycosylated Hemoglobin (HbA1c)

Hemoglobin is a red pigment responsible for carrying oxygen in red blood cells. It consists of four subunits, each containing a heme group conjugated with a polypeptide. In adults, the primary form of hemoglobin is **Hemoglobin A (HbA)**, which has two alpha (α) chains and two beta (β) chains.

What is HbA1c?

HbA1c is a glycosylated form of hemoglobin where glucose binds irreversibly to the beta chains. It reflects the average blood glucose levels over the past 2–3 months.

- **Normal Range**: 4–6% (average ~5%).
- **Clinical Significance**: Increased HbA1c levels indicate poor glycemic control and a higher risk of diabetes complications.

Advantages of HbA1c Testing

1. No need for fasting.
2. Greater stability compared to plasma glucose measurements.
3. Fewer day-to-day variations in results.
4. Strong correlation with the risk of hyperglycemic complications.

HbA1c as a Diagnostic Tool

In 2010, the ADA officially incorporated HbA1c as a diagnostic criterion for diabetes.

- **HbA1c ≥6.5%**: Diagnostic for diabetes.
- **HbA1c 5.7–6.4%**: Indicates **pre-diabetes**.
- **HbA1c 5.5–6%**: Individuals in this range are at **3–8 times higher risk** of developing diabetes in the future.

Estimated Average Glucose (eAG)

The following formula converts HbA1c values into estimated average glucose levels:

eAG (mg/dL) = 28.7 x HbA1c - 46.7

Limitations of HbA1c Testing

While HbA1c testing offers many advantages, it has some limitations:

1. **Interference from Abnormal Hemoglobins**: Certain hemoglobin variants can affect the accuracy of results.
2. **Red Blood Cell Lifespan**: Conditions like hemolytic anemia, chronic malaria, or recent blood transfusions can alter HbA1c levels.
3. **Age-Related Increases**: HbA1c levels may rise with age, independent of glucose metabolism.
4. **Ethnic Variations**: Minor racial and ethnic differences in HbA1c levels may exist.
5. **Not Suitable for Gestational Diabetes**: HbA1c is not recommended for diagnosing diabetes during pregnancy.

CHAPTER 5: The Role of Exercise in Diabetes

The Effect of Exercise on Diabetes

Obesity and reduced physical activity are two key factors that exacerbate diabetes. Numerous studies have established a strong relationship between:

- **Body weight gain**,
- **Obesity**,
- **Physical inactivity**,
- **Increased caloric intake**,

…and the rising prevalence of diabetes and coronary artery disease.

In both rural and urban populations, sedentary lifestyles significantly contribute to the increased prevalence of diabetes. By contrast, regular physical activity and exercise have been shown to reduce the incidence and control risk factors for diabetes.

The Role of Exercise in Diabetes Prevention and Management

Lifestyle Changes Over Medication

In the prevention and management of chronic diseases like diabetes and coronary artery disease, **lifestyle modifications** are often more effective than drug therapy. Exercise and physical activity are universally recommended as part of a healthy lifestyle for individuals across all age groups.

Expert Insights

Health and sports science experts emphasize the profound impact of regular physical activity on reducing the incidence and mortality associated with diabetes and cardiovascular diseases. By increasing energy expenditure, exercise helps:

1. **Control Hyperglycemia**: Improves blood sugar levels.
2. **Enhance Insulin Sensitivity**: Reduces insulin resistance in target tissues.
3. **Promote Weight Management**: Aids in weight loss and prevents obesity.
4. **Improve Cardiovascular Health**: Reduces the risk of heart-related complications.

Types, Intensity, and Duration of Exercise

The benefits of exercise depend on the **type**, **intensity**, and **duration** of physical activity. Tailored exercise programs can produce favorable effects on blood sugar control, overall fitness, and well-being in diabetic individuals.

Significance of Physical Activity in Diabetes Prevention

Increased physical activity and structured exercise programs are crucial for:

- **Primary Prevention**: Reducing the risk of developing diabetes in at-risk individuals.
- **Secondary Prevention**: Managing blood sugar levels and minimizing complications in those already diagnosed with diabetes.

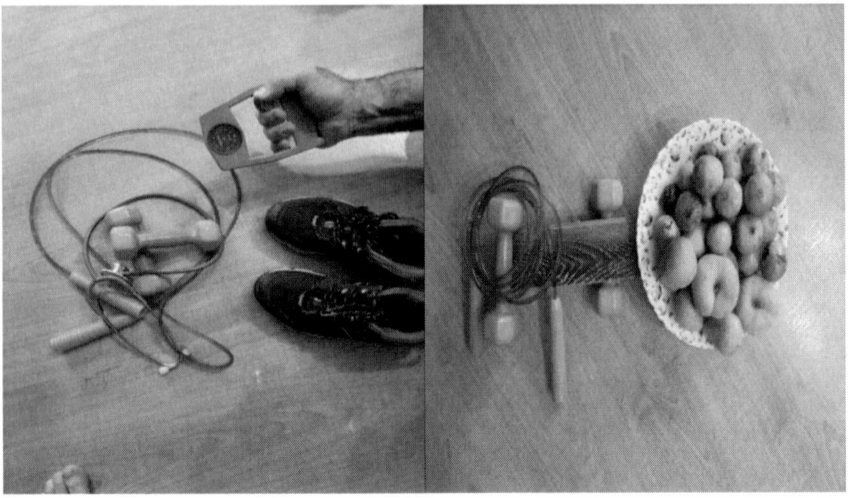

Figure 5: The Role of Physical Activity and Nutrition in Diabetes Prevention and Treatment.

Apolipoproteins and Their Role in Diabetes and Coagulation

Apolipoproteins

Apolipoproteins are proteins that bind to lipids (fats and cholesterol) to form **lipoproteins**, which transport fats through the blood, cerebrospinal fluid, and lymph. They play a critical role in lipid metabolism and are categorized into several classes and subclasses, including:

1. **Apolipoprotein A** (apoA1, apoA2, apoA4, apoA5)
2. **Apolipoprotein B** (apoB48, apoB100)
3. **Apolipoprotein C** (apoC-I, apoC-II, apoC-III, apoC-IV)
4. **Apolipoprotein D**
5. **Apolipoprotein E**
6. **Apolipoprotein F**
7. **Apolipoprotein H**

8. **Apolipoprotein L**
9. **Apolipoprotein M**

Apolipoproteins and Diabetes

- Studies show that the concentration of **lipoprotein A** is significantly higher in individuals with diabetes compared to non-diabetics.
- Research involving 210 type 2 diabetic patients revealed elevated levels of lipoprotein A and other lipids compared to 46 non-diabetic participants. After blood sugar control, these lipid levels decreased significantly.
- Increased lipoprotein A levels are also observed in diabetic individuals with cardiovascular complications.

Effect of Exercise on Apolipoproteins

- Endurance and resistance exercises significantly increase the levels of **Apolipoprotein A1 (ApoA1)** compared to inactive individuals.
- Improved lipid profiles and reduced cardiovascular risks are observed in physically active diabetic patients.

Aging, Coagulation, and Diabetes

Risks of Aging and Coagulation

Aging is a well-known risk factor for cardiovascular diseases, with evidence showing an increased prevalence of thrombotic conditions in older adults. Aging affects the **fibrinolytic system**, which is responsible for breaking down blood clots. Key findings include:

- Increased levels of **Plasminogen Activator Inhibitor-1 (PAI-1)** with aging, obesity, and inflammation.

- PAI-1 plays a critical role in thrombosis and atherosclerosis, and its deficiency is associated with bleeding.
- Psychological stress, insulin resistance, and obesity are additional factors that elevate PAI-1 levels, contributing to cardiovascular risks.

Fibrinolysis and Its Clinical Significance

Fibrinolysis is the process by which the body dissolves blood clots. Two key enzymes involved in this process are:

1. **Tissue Plasminogen Activator (t-PA)**: Converts plasminogen to plasmin, breaking down fibrin clots.
2. **Plasminogen Activator Inhibitor-1 (PAI-1)**: Inhibits t-PA, reducing fibrinolytic activity.

Impact of Obesity and Physical Activity on Coagulation

- Obesity, insulin resistance, and hypertension elevate PAI-1 levels, increasing the risk of thrombotic and cardiovascular diseases.
- Regular aerobic exercise reduces PAI-1 levels and enhances fibrinolytic activity, mitigating cardiovascular risks.

Physical Activity and Blood Coagulation in Diabetics

The Role of Exercise in Coagulation and Fibrinolysis

Regular physical activity improves fibrinolytic capacity and reduces coagulation factors. Studies have shown:

- Long-term aerobic training decreases PAI-1 levels and fibrinogen in healthy and diabetic individuals.
- Exercise increases the secretion of **t-PA**, accelerating clot dissolution and preventing thrombosis.

- Increased consumption of fruits and vegetables, which are rich in antioxidants, further protects against atherosclerosis and thrombosis.

Metabolic Benefits of Physical Activity

Brown Fat and Increased Metabolism

- Physical training induces the conversion of white adipose tissue into **brown adipose tissue**, which plays a thermogenic role due to its high mitochondrial density.
- Brown fat levels are inversely related to body mass index (BMI) and fat percentage, making it a critical factor in metabolic health.
- **Irisin**, a myokine released during exercise, promotes the browning of white fat and increases thermogenesis via the **FNDC5 gene** and **Uncoupling Protein-1 (UCP1)**.

Muscle Mass and Diabetes

Diabetes is associated with muscle mass loss (atrophy) due to:

- Increased protein breakdown and reduced synthesis.
- Low insulin levels, reduced IGF-1, and elevated cortisol levels.

Exercise and Muscle Preservation

- Exercise activates the **PI3K/Akt pathway**, inhibiting the muscle-degrading protein FOXO, thus preventing atrophy.
- Increased levels of **Peroxisome Proliferator-Activated Receptor-γ Coactivator 1-α (PGC1α)** in muscles reduce protein degradation and support muscle preservation.

CHAPTER 6: Diabetes and Heart Tissue

Physical Exercise and Apoptosis in Heart Tissue

Apoptosis, or programmed cell death, plays a significant role in various cardiac disorders. Two key proteins regulate this process:

- **Bcl-2**: An anti-apoptotic protein that protects heart cells by inhibiting cell death.
- **Bax**: A pro-apoptotic protein that induces apoptosis during cellular stress or damage.

Excessive expression of Bax is strongly associated with cell death, while increased Bcl-2 levels enhance cell survival.

Impact of Exercise on Apoptosis

- Intense physical activity may temporarily increase apoptosis rates.
- Moderate and continuous exercise, however, has been shown to reduce apoptosis in various tissues, including the heart.
- Regular exercise mitigates cellular aging, a key contributor to physiological decline in diabetes, and promotes healthy cell function in the heart, brain, and body.

Aerobic Training and Diabetic Cardiomyopathy

Benefits of Aerobic Exercise on Cardiac Function

Aerobic exercise improves heart health by:

1. Reducing the risk of cardiovascular diseases.
2. Enhancing heart function through **physiological hypertrophy**, which includes:

- Structural changes in the heart.
- Increased expression of cardiac hypertrophy genes.
- Improved myocardial function and metabolism.

What is Diabetic Cardiomyopathy?

Diabetic cardiomyopathy refers to abnormalities in the myocardium caused by diabetes, leading to:

- Coronary artery disease.
- Hypertension.
- Valvular heart disease.

Prevalence:

- Diabetic women: 5 times higher risk of heart failure.
- Diabetic men: 2.4 times higher risk of heart failure.

Early Characteristics:

- Left ventricular hypertrophy.
- Fibrosis.
- Cell signaling dysfunction.

Aerobic Training, Lipid Profile, and Insulin Resistance

Lipid Disorders in Diabetes

Diabetes often involves lipid abnormalities, including:

- Increased levels of total cholesterol (TC), low-density lipoprotein (LDL), and triglycerides (TG).
- Reduced levels of high-density lipoprotein (HDL).

These changes increase the risk of atherosclerosis, even in cases where lipid profiles appear normal, due to altered apolipoproteins.

Role of ApoA-I

- ApoA-I is the main protein in HDL, comprising 70% of its protein mass.
- It plays a critical role in reverse cholesterol transport, slowing atherosclerosis progression.

Effects of Exercise

- Studies show that regular physical activity:
    - Improves lipid profiles.
    - Reduces insulin resistance and increases insulin sensitivity.
    - Increases circulating levels of ApoA-I, aiding in cholesterol management.

Aerobic Exercise and GLUT2 in Diabetes

The Role of GLUT2 in Glucose Metabolism

GLUT2, a glucose transporter, plays a crucial role in pancreatic β-cell function and blood sugar regulation. Dysregulation of GLUT2 is associated with:

- Impaired glucose transport.
- β-cell dysfunction.
- Increased risk of type 2 diabetes.

Impact of High-Fat Diets

- High-fat diets contribute to insulin resistance, β-cell senescence, and reduced β-cell proliferation, leading to glucose intolerance and type 2 diabetes.

Benefits of Aerobic Exercise

Endurance training improves:

1. **Insulin Sensitivity**: Enhances glucose uptake and utilization.
2. **Pancreatic Function**: Reduces glucose and fat toxicity in β-cells.
3. **Oxidative Capacity**: Increases mitochondrial content and oxidative enzyme activity in skeletal muscle.
4. **β-cell Health**: Decreases inflammation and oxidative stress, improving function and regeneration of pancreatic cells.

Regular exercise also restores the function of GLUT2 and GLUT4, essential for maintaining blood sugar homeostasis.

Aerobic exercise plays a vital role in mitigating the cardiac and metabolic complications of diabetes. From reducing apoptosis in heart tissues to improving lipid profiles, insulin sensitivity, and β-cell function, exercise is an effective strategy for managing diabetes and promoting heart health.

This revised chapter provides clear sections and logical flow, ensuring the information is accessible and engaging. Let me know if you'd like additional refinements or expansions!

CHAPTER 7: Diabetes and Nutrition

The Role of Nutrition in Diabetes

The food we consume significantly impacts the body's physiological functions. Dietary choices can either aid in managing diabetes or worsen its complications. Below are the key nutritional considerations for individuals with diabetes:

Dietary Fibers

Dietary fibers are essential for improving digestion, regulating blood sugar levels, and lowering cholesterol. Types of dietary fibers and their benefits include:

1. **Cellulose (e.g., whole wheat, cereal brand, vegetables)**:
    - Increases water retention in the body.
    - Adds bulk to stools, reducing the risk of tumors.
2. **Pectin (e.g., apples, strawberries, carrots, citrus fruits)**:
    - Promotes lipid excretion.
    - Reduces serum cholesterol levels.
3. **Gums (e.g., barley, beans)**:
    - Forms a gel-like substance that slows digestion and glucose absorption.
4. **Fructans (e.g., inulin found in chicory and onion)**:
    - Acts as a prebiotic, stimulating the growth of beneficial gut bacteria.
5. **Synthetic Compounds (e.g., sorbitol)**:
    - Can replace sugar and act as stool bulkers.

The Importance of Fruits

Fruits are rich in water, vitamins, minerals, and dietary fiber, offering several health benefits, including detoxification and improved digestion. However, certain fruits that are high in sugar, such as dates and dried figs, may not be suitable for diabetic patients due to their rapid sugar absorption.

Synergistic Effects of Exercise and Vitamins

1. **Vitamin C**:
    - When combined with physical activity, vitamin C helps prevent and treat diabetes.
2. **Vitamin E**:
    - Beneficial for managing diabetes, cardiovascular diseases, and skin disorders.

The Role of Weight Management

- A weight reduction of even 5% can significantly improve blood sugar control and lower the risk of type 2 diabetes.
- A balanced diet and regular physical activity are crucial for diabetes prevention and management.

Diabetes and Diet Plan

Proteins

Proteins from sources such as chicken, eggs, fish, nuts, and legumes are crucial for blood sugar regulation. They induce satiety, reducing carbohydrate consumption and sugar absorption.

Healthy Carbohydrates

Carbohydrates are converted into glucose during digestion, so choosing the right types is essential.

- **Recommended Sources**:
    - Fruits, vegetables, whole grains, legumes (e.g., beans, lentils), and low-fat dairy products.
- **To Avoid**:
    - Sugary drinks, sweets, processed foods, and refined sugars.

Good Fats

Unsaturated fats can lower cholesterol levels and support heart health. Examples include:

- **Sources**:
  - Avocados, nuts (e.g., almonds, walnuts, pistachios), canola oil, and olive oil.
- **Note**: Avoid excessive consumption, as these fats are calorie-dense.

Medicinal Plants for Diabetes Management

The use of medicinal plants is gaining attention for their role in managing diabetes. Below are some of the most effective plants:

1. **Garlic**:
   - Contains compounds such as **allicin, allixin, and ajoene**, which have antifungal, antiparasitic, antiplatelet, and antibiotic effects.
   - Rich in vitamins (A, B, C), selenium, and zinc, garlic has been shown to:
     - Lower blood pressure.
     - Reduce serum glucose, triglycerides, and cholesterol levels.
     - Act as an anticancer agent.
   - A study revealed that alcoholic extracts of garlic significantly decreased glucose, triglycerides, cholesterol, and liver enzyme levels (Figure 6).

Proper nutrition is fundamental in managing diabetes. Combining a balanced diet with regular physical activity and incorporating medicinal plants and vitamins can help regulate blood sugar levels, improve overall health, and reduce complications.

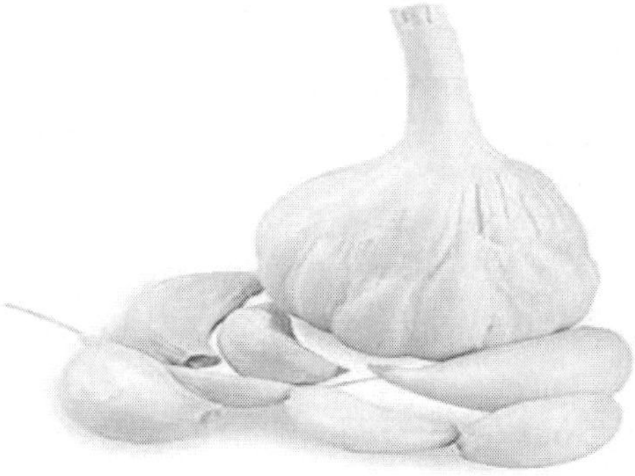

Figure 6. Garlic and control of diabetes

1. Cinnamon

Cinnamon bark is widely used as a spice and has demonstrated effectiveness in managing diabetes. Studies confirm that cinnamon:

- Reduces fasting serum glucose levels (Figure 7).
- May have benefits for patients with immunodeficiency diseases such as HIV.

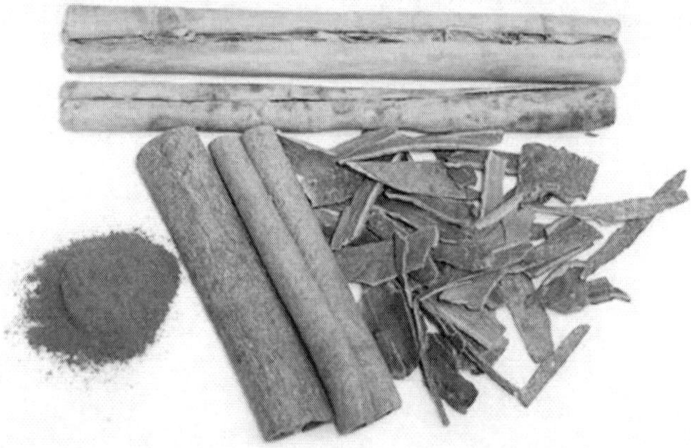

Figure 7: Cinnamon and its role in controlling diabetes.

2. Mespilus

Extracts from the leaves of Mespilus (commonly known as medlar) have shown significant blood glucose-lowering effects. Mechanisms include:

- Increased insulin secretion.
- Enhanced glucose transport via insulin-dependent pathways.
- Antioxidant properties from flavonoids, which prevent lipid peroxidation (Figure 8).

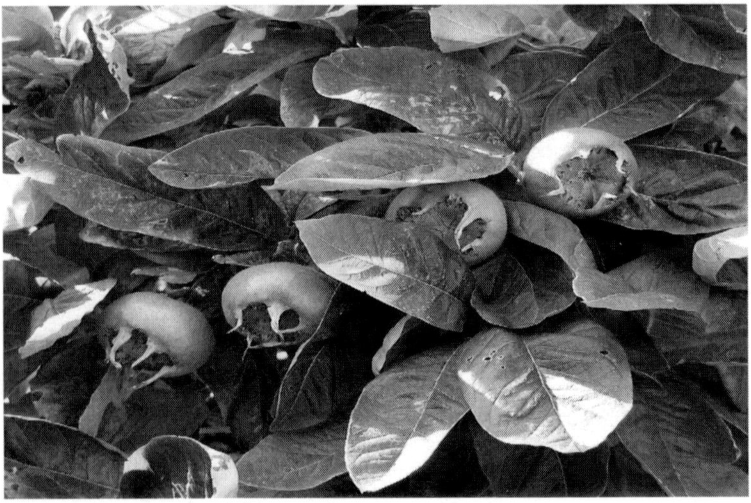

Figure 8: Mespilus and its role in controlling diabetes.

3. Cuminum Cyminum (Cumin)

Cumin seeds are rich in antioxidants, including ascorbic acid, niacin, copper, and magnesium. These compounds contribute to:

- Anti-diabetic effects.
- Improved glycemic control (Figure 9).

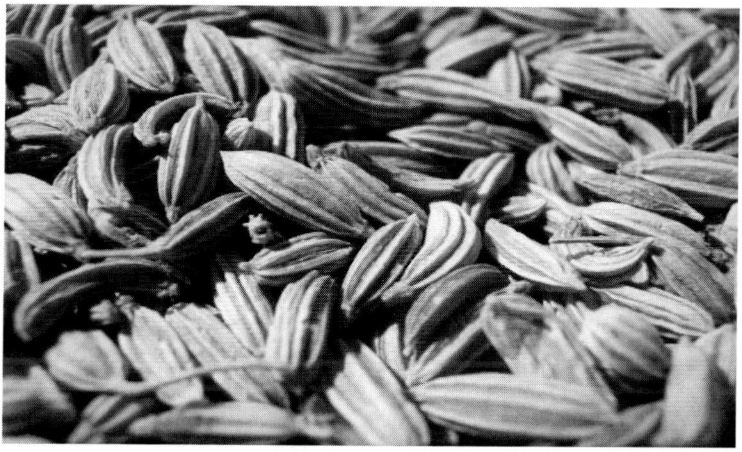

Figure 9: Cuminum Cyminum and its role in controlling diabetes.

4. Citrullus Colocynthis (Bitter Apple)

The chemical compounds in bitter apple, such as saponins, flavonoids, and glycosides, aid in diabetes management by:

- Reducing fasting blood sugar levels and HbA1c over two months of usage.
- Stimulating beta cells in the pancreas to release more insulin (Figure 10).

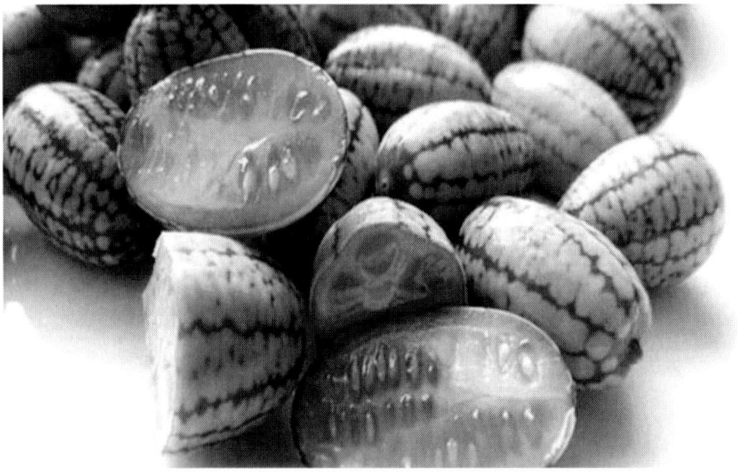

Figure 10: Citrullus Colocynthis and its role in controlling diabetes.

5. Fenugreek

Fenugreek seeds and extracts offer several anti-diabetic benefits:

- Enhancing glucose entry into muscle cells.
- Reducing carbohydrate absorption from the intestine.
- Lowering blood glucose and cholesterol levels in type 1 and type 2 diabetic patients (Figure 11).

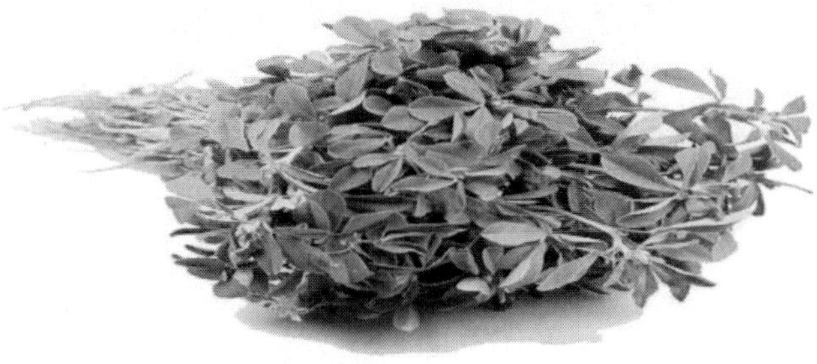

Figure 11: Fenugreek and its role in controlling diabetes.

6. Silybum (Milk Thistle)

Milk thistle seeds and extracts are effective for:

- Reducing insulin resistance.
- Lowering blood glucose, HbA1c, and cholesterol levels.
- Acting as a strong antioxidant, protecting against oxidative stress and lipid peroxidation (Figure 12).

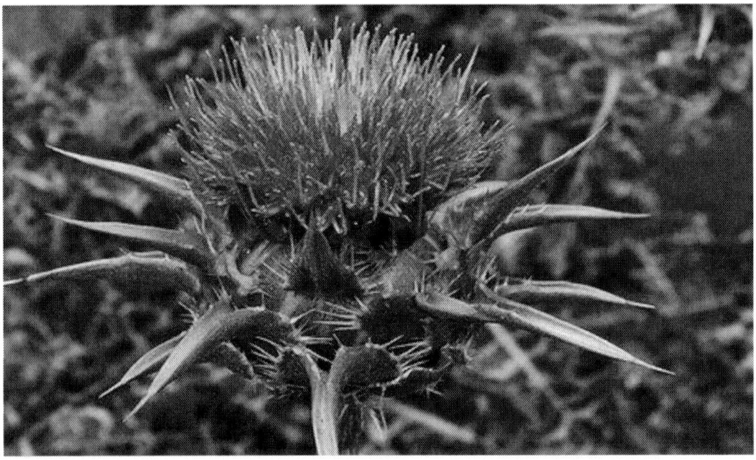

Figure 12: Silybum and its role in controlling diabetes.

7. Green Tea

Green tea offers numerous benefits for diabetic patients:

- Increases insulin levels.
- Lowers glucose, fatty acid, and triglyceride levels.
- Improves insulin resistance by increasing GLUT4 expression (Figure 13).

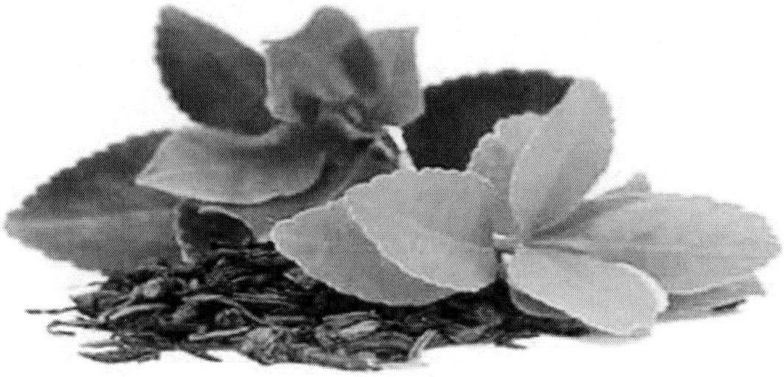

Figure 13: Green tea and its role in controlling diabetes.

8. Vaccinium (Bilberry)

Bilberry fruits and leaves regulate blood glucose levels by:

- Reducing HbA1c and fasting glucose.
- Increasing blood insulin levels (Figure 14).

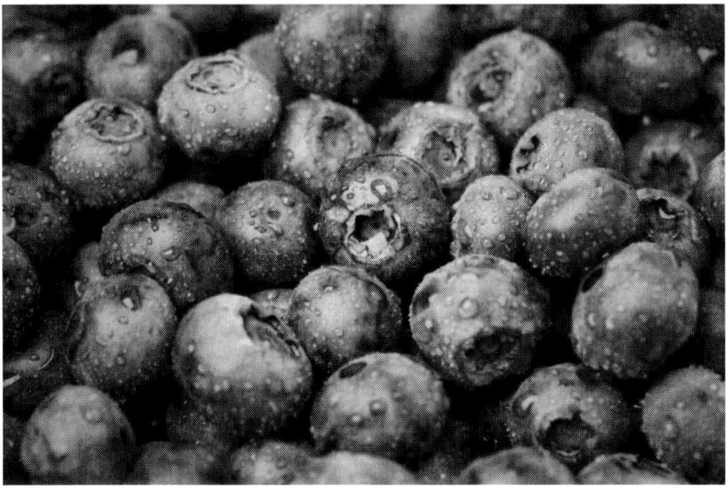

Figure 14: Vaccinium and its role in controlling diabetes.

9. Sweet Potato

Rich in antioxidants, sweet potatoes:

- Regulate blood sugar levels.
- Lower the risk of heart disease, diabetes, and obesity.
- Improve digestion and boost immune function (Figure 15).

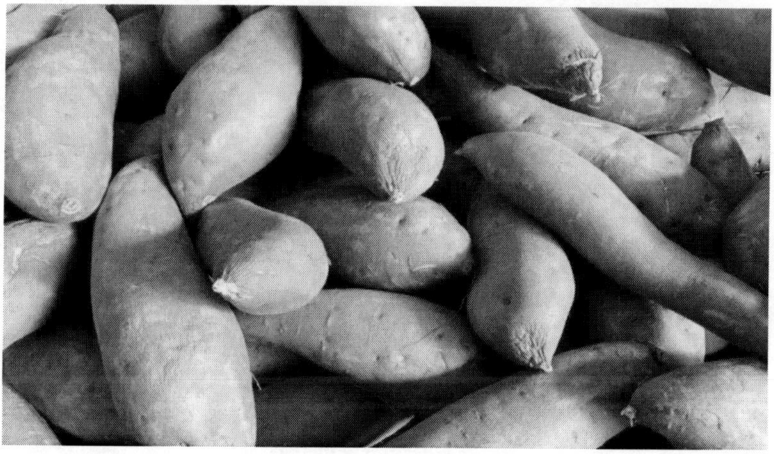

Figure 15: Sweet potato and its role in controlling diabetes.

10. Walnut

Walnuts help in diabetes management by:

- Reducing insulin resistance.
- Stabilizing blood sugar levels with their high fiber content (Figure 16).

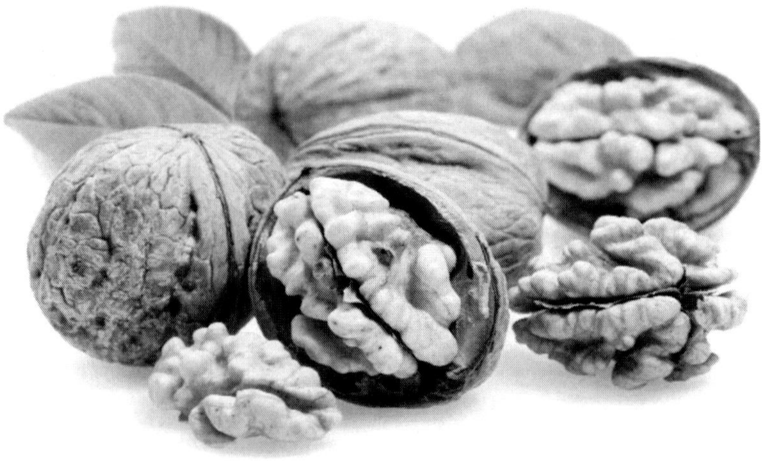

Figure 16: Walnut and its role in controlling diabetes.

11. Pomegranate

Pomegranate components (juice, seeds, and peel) provide:

- Antioxidant and anti-inflammatory benefits.
- Blood sugar reduction by inhibiting cortisol and catecholamine release.
- Cardiovascular protection by preventing angiotensin II activity (Figure 17).

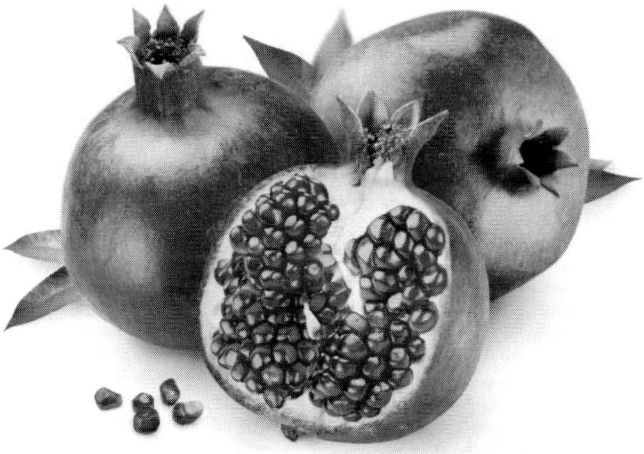

Figure 17: Pomegranate and its role in controlling diabetes.

12. Bitter Cucumber (Bitter Melon)

Bitter cucumber supports diabetes treatment by:

- Enhancing insulin secretion and beta-cell protection.
- Regulating intestinal glucose transport.
- Activating AMP-activated protein kinase (AMPK), which improves insulin sensitivity (Figure 18).

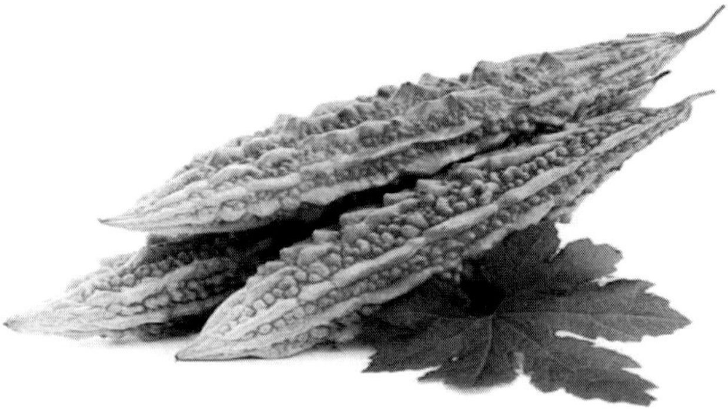

Figure 18: Bitter cucumber and its role in controlling diabetes.

13. Nettle

Nettle extracts, derived from its leaves, roots, and seeds, have protective effects against:

- Elevated blood glucose.
- Pancreatic cell damage.
- Cardiovascular risks, by improving heart rate and blood pressure control (Figure 19).

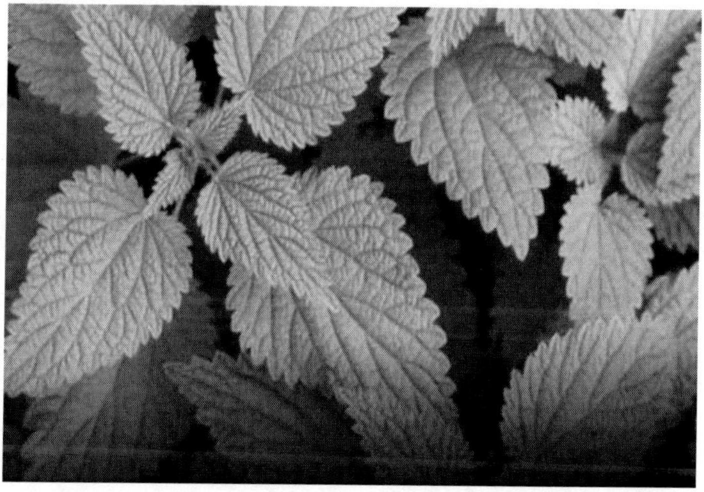

Figure 19: Nettle and its role in controlling diabetes.

The integration of medicinal plants into diabetes care offers a complementary approach to managing blood sugar levels and preventing complications. Along with proper diet and exercise, these natural remedies can enhance the quality of life for diabetic patients.

Made in United States
North Haven, CT
03 November 2026

21729489R00030